THE NINE HOUR
NEW YOU

MIRANDA LLEWELLYN

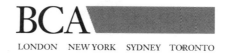

BCA

LONDON   NEW YORK   SYDNEY   TORONTO

ADVICE TO THE READER

Before following any exercise or dietary advice contained in this book, it is recommended that you consult your doctor if you suffer from any health problems or special conditions or are in any doubt as to its suitability.

FOR ROSS

This edition published in 1996 by BCA by arrangement with Boxtree Limited

Copyright © Miranda Llewellyn

The right of Miranda Llewellyn to be identified as Author of this work has been asserted by her in accordance with the Copyright, Designs and Patents Act 1988

Flex-a-Band and the Flex-a-Band logo are trademarks of Medisport International Ltd

1 3 5 7 9 10 8 6 4 2

CN 3195

Text design by DW Design, London

Cover design by Shoot That Tiger!
All exercise photography by Damien Walker

Cartoons by Kate Taylor
Line drawings by Raymond Turvey
Clothing and shoes supplied by L.A. Gear

Printed and bound in Great Britain by The Bath Press

A CIP catalogue entry for this book
is available from the British Library

CONTENTS

INTRODUCTION

Over the many years that I have been teaching exercise, I have heard the same problems over and over again:

- 'I eat hardly anything, but I'm still putting on weight.'

- 'I don't have time to exercise.'

- 'What can I do about my hips/bum/tum/thighs?'

- 'I was on a strict diet last year, but since I stopped I'm bigger than ever.'

The list goes on and I'm sure it's familiar to you too.

The secret to having a shapely, toned body is neither crash or fad diets (especially not meal-replacement drinks), nor exercise regimes that half kill you; it is a much easier, gentler approach.
Most people know by now that exercise and diet are what keep you in shape – sounds good in theory, but in practice no one really explains how much to eat, when and what in relation to exercise. Once you get the combination right the rest is simple and, what's more, **it works!**

You don't need to feel that keeping in shape is a huge task, continually put off because you're so busy that you just can't face it. Keep calm – you don't need to spend a fortune on expensive club memberships or equipment, or devote hours of your time to the gym.

The Nine Hour New You is a programme designed to show results in double-quick time with a minimum of effort. In addition, once you've got into the swing of it, you should be able to maintain the lifestyle changes for the rest of your life, and never worry about your figure again.

LOOKING AT YOURSELF: A PERSONAL NOTE

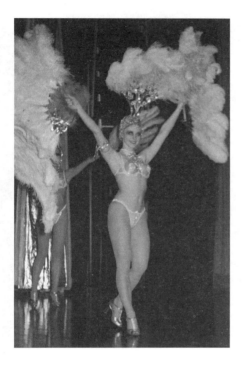

Before I started my fitness consultancy, I was a professional dancer. When I started my dancer's training – which was very rigorous – it was drummed into me that I should never, ever get fat. The pressure on me and my contemporaries to be thin, thinner, thinnest was tremendous – with always the threat that we would not find work if we were not.

At 5'8" tall with a large frame and a

naturally muscular build it should have been obvious that I was never going to fit into a size 8 dress. But this became one of my greatest ambitions, and pursuing it with a kind of religious fervour, I turned to a strict starvation diet to achieve this unattainable goal.

Every day I went through my paces in front of a mirror, dressed in a figure-hugging leotard and tights, ostensibly to correct my technique, but more often than not to have a silent conversation with myself about my shape, criticising each bump and bulge, imaginary or otherwise.

This negative and damaging attitude continued into my working life as a dancer, where not only was my body continually under scrutiny, but also I felt all the insecurities a woman often feels about the way she looks being magnified by the unforgiving spotlight. My whole career and livelihood hinged on my appearance.

And no-one ever encouraged me to think otherwise about my body. To the contrary: I remember once going for a costume fitting where the seamstress accidentally jabbed a pin into my hip. 'OW!,' I yelled, my eyes smarting. 'Well, luvvie,' she said, 'just a little hint that you need to lose some blubber. A few stone should do it.' A few stone?! I only weighed **9** stone!

However, these days I'm over a stone heavier – but a dress size smaller.

When I worked at the Moulin Rouge in Paris in 1975, the standards were high. Comments made during rehearsals such as 'We'll put the fat ones at the back' did little to help my self-esteem or body image (although in spite of this the back row had no shortage of 'stage door Johnnies' – quite the opposite, in fact).

1975 was also the year in which a major French fashion designer modelled his whole collection using transvestites. At about this time I began to question the ideals that had been drummed into me. What about real women? Why were women being indoctrinated into believing that to be glamorous or attractive or feminine you had to aspire to an impossible ideal, and one that was often injurious to both physical and mental health?

It's interesting to note that ideals change from country to country. And you don't have to go as far as Tonga (where size is a measure of beauty) to find the difference: when I was first accepted as a Bluebell Girl it was decided that I shouldn't work in Paris as I was too short and stocky; I was to be sent to Spain, where my shape was considered very attractive.

It was after the birth of my first child in 1982 that I began to teach fitness classes. I started to come into contact with literally hundreds of women who poured their hearts out to me about their figure problems. However they usually finished up by saying, 'But you don't have to worry though, do you?'

Wow, talk about understatement – I'd done enough worrying over the years to last me a lifetime!

So over the years, both by coming to understand my own body and through teaching many others, my philosophy and outlook has changed considerably. Now I know that bodies respond well to tender loving care. Don't punish your body by starving it, overworking it or generally mistreating it, and above all don't transmit or take on board negative mental messages. Treat your body as you would your best friend – be kind to it and consider its needs – it will respond by not letting you down.

Exercise and healthy eating are part of the way to achieve the New You. But you'd also be amazed at how looking at yourself in a new way will help you to achieve your goals – it's a very important part of **The Nine Hour New You.**

THE NINE HOUR NEW YOU PROGRAMME

This programme is geared to six weeks at 1.5 hours per week as follows:
- **20 minutes walking**
- **followed by 10 minutes body toning**
- **3 times per week.**

In only nine hours you can have a New You!

The Walking Programme is a cheap, effective, easy and pleasant way to incorporate aerobic activity into your daily life. Not only is it great for inch loss, but also for a healthy heart and increased bone density. It can be fun as well if you do it with your friends – if you do, make sure that you share the same goals.

To enable you to do the toning part of the programme, **Firm 'n' Fit While You Sit** and **Terrific Toning**, enclosed with this book is a **Flex-a-Band**, which, because it works on the principle of resistance, means that you see results in a fraction of the time normally required. For instance, where you would normally need to do 2 sets of 8 repetitions of stomach crunches, by using the Flex-a-Band you would only need to do 1 set of 8 repetitions for the same result, which equals less time spent on exercising, more

time to enjoy the results. If you do not do the body toning after the walking but wish to split the programme, e.g. Monday – walk 20 minutes, Tuesday – body toning 10 minutes, this is fine, but you must include a 5-minute warm up before you start the body toning.

In the **Food File** chapter I have included healthy eating guidelines and explained, as simply as I know how, the effects of various foods on the body.

REMEMBER
A diet is temporary; healthy eating is for life

A number of features have been used in this book to help you get the most out of this programme. Each exercise has clear step-by-step instructions and one or more photographs to illustrate the correct body

REPETITION = The performance of an exercise

SET = How many times you need to repeat that exercise

position. Positioning to avoid is also illustrated by photographs, marked with a large cross. Body check boxes also help with this. It is important to position your body correctly and carry out the exercise movements as instructed to benefit fully from the programme and to avoid injury. The exercises each conclude with a box detailing the required number of repetitions of each movement and of each exercise as a whole, and listing the sequence of movements to be counted through the exercise. Count slowly as shown in the boxes at the front of each set of exercises.

 2 in 1 flashes indicate where two parts of your body benefit from one exercise.

Smiling and frowning faces indicate things you can do to help or hinder your New You Programme.

Definition boxes help with additional information.

Start by reading **Understanding Your Body** and **Mastering the Technique to a New You**. The latter features a suggested week-by-week exercise plan for the entire programme and provides blank **Body Plan** charts for you to keep a record of your exercises and walks. Following this is a **Figure Fact** chart for you to monitor your progress each week by measuring key body sites. These results will encourage you to persevere!

Read the **Using the Flex-a-Band** chapter before starting the toning exercises to ensure correct technique and safety.

Begin with the **Walking Programme**, and follow this with the Flex-a-Band exercises.

Try the Firm 'n' Fit While You Sit exercises if you are unused to exercising; within a fortnight you will be able to move on to the **Terrific Toning** exercises for maximum effect.

Remember to ask your doctor for the thumbs up before you start this or any other exercise programme.

If you have worked out at a gym or attended a fitness class you may find you are familiar with some of the exercises in this book. Performed properly, with the Flex-a-Band, these exercises are much better!

It doesn't matter in which order you attempt these exercises – they have been designed for you to pick and mix those you prefer to make the programme as fun and as painless as possible. You will be able to do more as you improve. Do remember, however, that it is essential to carry out the instructions warming up and cooling every time you exercise.

Although this workout programme has been designed and written for women, men are welcome to follow the programme; but they may find it is less effective for them. A similar programme aimed specifically at men is in the process of being developed.

Begin at the beginning and **ENJOY!**

UNDERSTANDING YOUR BODY

BODY SHAPING = balance between good nutrition, strength and aerobic training

Betty Bumwiggle realizes that her curves have become excessively abundant – yet again! In a wild panic, she starts a drastic diet and flings herself into an over-enthusiastic, not to mention painful, exercise programme.

1 week later: she's knackered, bad tempered, and everything **HURTS!** She gives up the exercise and just continues the diet.

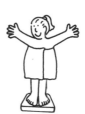

2 weeks later: the scales show she's lost a few pounds – YIPPEE! BUT everything seems so wobbly and saggy – **YEUCH!**

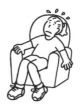

3 weeks later: she gives up.

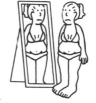

4 weeks later: Now how did that happen? She's even curvier than she was a month ago – not to mention wallowing in the depths of gloom and despair.

This is an all too familiar situation. Betty tried to work her body at an unaccustomed level with insufficient food fuels; when she got tired and her muscles 'complained', she stopped the exercise. Sustained exercise is the key to inch loss.

PROPER FOOD INTAKE = the energy needed to perform sustained exercise

TIPS

1 Throw away your scales – yes, really. Who cares how much you weigh if you're a size 12 (or 14, or 16, or whatever you want to be)?
THINK ABOUT IT.

2 Don't fall into the trap of 'being good' or 'being naughty'. You can eat whatever you like as long as you are aware of how certain foods will affect you. When you are aware of how they will affect you, you can make educated choices. Making educated choices = being in control of your own body.

3 Be kind to yourself – this probably sounds strange, but hundreds of women spend their lives being rude and unkind to themselves. How would you like it if someone kept telling you how much they hated you? Your body's much more likely to co-operate in working towards the **New You** if you're kind to it.

4 Have a realistic body image.

5 Refuse to conform to expected ideals – be yourself.

By the way, have you ever heard any of the following myths? Chances
are you have, and more than once at that.

READ AND MEMORISE THE TRUE FACTS

FALSE	TRUE
'If I strength train, when I stop the muscle will turn to fat.'	Fat and muscle are different substances, therefore fat cannot become muscle and muscle cannot become fat.
'I can sweat off pounds of fat in the sauna.'	The weight lost while in a sauna is primarily water and body fluids, and could well be damaging. Don't try to sweat off pounds; it could lead to dehydration or heat stroke.
'Spot reducing is the best way to trim your figure.'	A good zit lotion would work just as well! Seriously, you can exercise the muscle which is underneath the fat and, while that muscle can become nicely toned, to lose fat you need either to decrease your food intake or increase aerobic activity – or both.
'Weight problems run in my family, so I've got no chance.'	Although some people are undoubtedly born with genes that predispose them to gain weight, this does not mean that you have to follow in the family footsteps. Nutritional habits are formed very early in life, so there could well be an unbroken chain of bad eating patterns learned from one generation to another.
'I'm heavy because I have big bones.'	'Heavy' you may be, but 'fat' no, and I doubt that heavy bones could account for more than a couple of pounds of weight, certainly not inches of fat.
'I'm this size because I have water retention.'	Um – yes, sure, but five stone of it? (I don't think so.)

**Aerobic exercise is an excellent form of exercise for inch loss. This is a
way of conditioning the heart and lungs, using a variety of activities that
create an increased demand for oxygen over an extended period of time.**

BODY TYPES

There are just three basic body types:

Ectomorphs – Suzy Slynkily-Slim is an ectomorph; she has a lean, thin body.

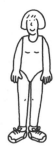

Mesomorphs – Mandy Musclemight is a mesomorph; she has clearly defined muscle on her shapely body.

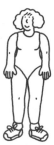

Endomorphs – Cherry Chubbington is an endomorph; she has a primarily round, chubby body – sometimes called 'cuddly'.

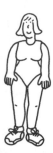

Just to complicate matters, there are many variations of these body types. Most people tend to be a blend of two classifications. For example, you could be a Cherry Musclemight, with a muscular, hefty build (mesomorphic endomorph). In case you wondered, this is my body type!

FACT   Muscle weighs more than fat

Whatever your body type, you can greatly improve your shape by good nutrition and exercise.

FAT – WHY, OH WHY IS IT THERE?

It's all down to gender. Men tend to put on weight in an 'apple' shape, and women in a 'pear' shape.

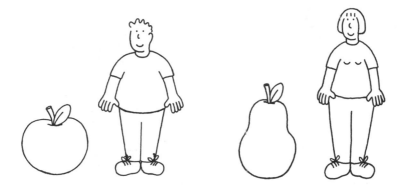

Question: FAT – What is it actually?

Answer: Quite simply, it is stored energy. If your fuel (calorie) intake exceeds your energy output, the difference is stored as fat.

Seems pretty simple really – if you do need to improve your shape either burn up the calories as you eat them, or don't put them into your system in the first place. If you're really in trouble and have vast reserves of stored calories (fat), try putting in fewer calories and taking extra exercise to use up the reserves.

Check the Food File section on pages 89–93 to see which foods contain the most fat.

FOOD FACT 1

Physically active people will burn more calories than inactive people (which means they can eat more without putting on weight).

FOOD FACT 2

Carbohydrates help make the body fuel needed for aerobic exercise. If the fuel in your body tank drops too low, you will be too tired to continue exercising.

MASTERING THE TECHNIQUE TO A NEW YOU

Good technique is vital to safe and effective exercise.

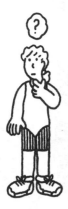

WHAT'S 'TECHNIQUE'?

> Technique is how well you perform an exercise, so that you gain the maximum physical benefits

BREATHING (PLEASE DO!!!)

Breathe evenly as you exercise; don't hold your breath – for obvious reasons. Try breathing out on the effort or hardest part, and in as you release.

PERFECT POSTURE

Believe it or not, quite apart from the fact that good posture is essential for getting the best results from your training and body development, it can also affect safety. If you try to work your muscles when you are out of alignment, it can result in injury. Also, have you ever heard the phrase 'looking like a victim'? This means quite simply that your body looks as if it is apologizing for being there. If you walk tall and proud you will also look visibly slimmer in seconds.

Take a look at the following seven photos:

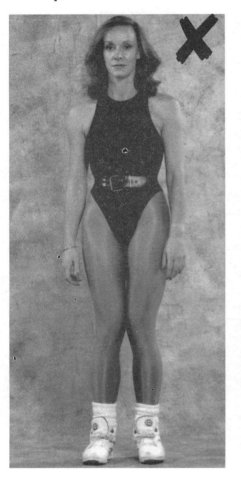

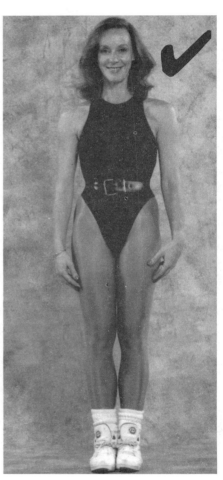

Note how my knees are 'knocking' together, putting severe strain on the joints. My hips are out of alignment, putting strain on my lower back, and my ribcage has dropped. Not one of my best snaps!

Much better.

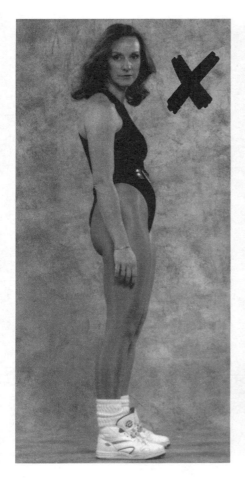

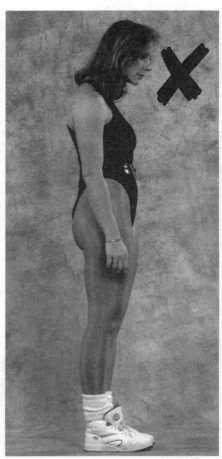

Note the rounded shoulders and dropped ribcage, which will affect my breathing capacity and, would you believe, my digestion as well.

My stomach is out because, with my hips pushed forwards, it is very difficult for it to do anything else! The droopy bum is a by-product of the position of my hips.

It looks like I've got the cares of the world on my shoulders. In later life I'll develop a 'dowager's hump'.

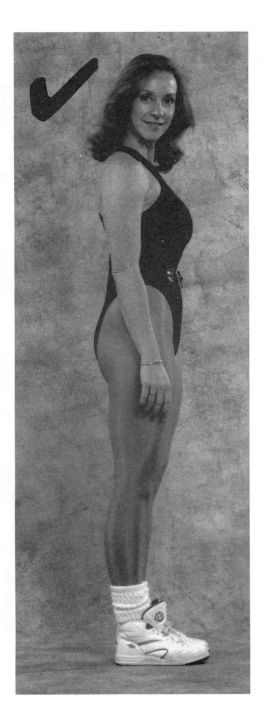

My shoulders are now in line with hips, ribcage lifted, tummy in – and bum is definitely better (well, almost!).

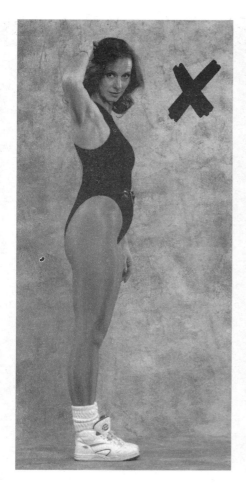

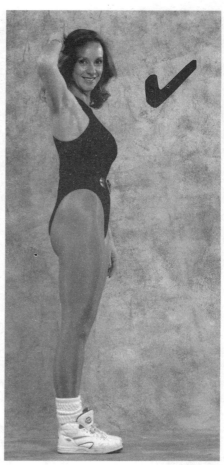

Oh boy! I'm going to have back problems if I keep arching my back like this.

Tailbone pulled down and tummy tight. Instant improvement and I didn't sweat a drop!

Ten tall 'n' trim tips

1 Keep your head up and 'centred'. Don't push it forward.

2 Relax your shoulders and neck.

3 Keep your ribcage lifted and shoulders back and down.

4 Consciously lengthen your spine.

5 Pull down with your tailbone and in with your tummy.

6 Don't allow your pelvis to push forward.

7 Keep your hips in line with your knees.

8 Keep your knees in line with your ankles.

9 When standing, your weight should be very slightly over the balls of your feet.

10 Don't allow the arches of your feet to drop.

FACT FILE　　Did you know?

● Most injuries associated with exercise can be blamed on poor body alignment.

● Bad posture can affect your digestion.

● Slouching can affect your lung capacity.

● If you stand badly you are more susceptible to backache and headaches.

● Good posture can improve your sex life!

By the way: Stretching is a great way to help re-align your body. Take a look at the stretches on pages 83 - 88.

DON'T EAT JUST BEFORE EXERCISING

When you work out your muscles will put in a demand for extra blood. If this happens, any food left in your stomach will just stay there and can make you feel sick.

But if you have eaten nothing for several hours before you exercise, you will probably feel tired and weak during your workout.

So what's the answer? Eat a light meal high in carbohydrates and low in protein and fat about two or three hours before your workout.

Why low in protein?
Because protein takes a long time to move through the digestive system.

Why low in fat?
Because fat will slow down your food's journey through the body.

So now you know!

Your body plan

On the following pages are suggested activity charts for your six-week exercise plan. These are followed by blank charts for you to complete for each week of your Nine Hour New You programme.

Your figure facts

● Measure yourself before you start the walking and toning programmes.

● Measure yourself each week.

● Try to measure each body site at exactly the same place each time.

● Measure either in inches or centimetres, whichever you prefer.

FIGURE FACT CHART

	BUST	UPPER ARMS	WAIST	HIPS	THIGHS
WEEK 1					
WEEK 2					
WEEK 3					
WEEK 4					
WEEK 5					
WEEK 6					

KEEP A RECORD!

C = CHAIR   F = FLOOR   S = STANDING

DAY	WALKING	SETS	UPPER BODY	SETS	LOWER BODY	TOTAL TIME
MONDAY	20 MINS	C2	BICEPS	C2	ABDOMINALS	30 MINS
		C2	TRICEPS (I each side)	C2	INNER THIGH	
		C2	PULL DOWN (I each side)	C2	OUTER THIGH	
		C2	CHEST PRESS	C2	QUADS (I on each leg)	
				C2	HAMSTRINGS (I on each leg)	
TUESDAY						
WEDNESDAY	20 MINS	S2	UPPER BACK	C2	ABDOMINALS	30 MINS
		S2	CHEST	C2	INNER THIGH	
		S2	BICEPS	C2	OUTER THIGH	
		S2	TRICEPS (I on each side)	C2	QUADS (I on each leg)	
				C2	HAMSTRINGS (I on each leg)	
THURSDAY						
FRIDAY						
SATURDAY	20 MINS	S4	UPPER BACK	F2	ABDOMINALS 1	30 MINS
		S4	CHEST			
		S1	BICEPS (I on each side)			
		S1	TRICEPS (I on each side)	F1	BACK	
				F2	INNER THIGH (I on each leg)	
				F2	OUTER THIGH	
SUNDAY						

DON'T FORGET TO STRETCH !

WEEK NO:1 **YOUR BODY PLAN**

C = CHAIR   F = FLOOR   S = STANDING

DAY	WALKING	SETS	UPPER BODY	SETS	LOWER BODY	TOTAL TIME
MONDAY						
TUESDAY						
WEDNESDAY						
THURSDAY						
FRIDAY						
SATURDAY						
SUNDAY						

DON'T FORGET TO STRETCH !

WEEK NO:2 **SUGGESTED BODY PLAN**

C = CHAIR   F = FLOOR   S = STANDING

DAY	WALKING	SETS	UPPER BODY	SETS	LOWER BODY	TOTAL TIME
MONDAY	20 MINS					20 MINS
TUESDAY		S1	BICEPS	F2	ABDOMINALS (1)	10 MINS
		S2	TRICEPS (I on each side)	F1	ABDOMINALS (3)	
				F1	BACK	
				F2	INNER THIGH (I each leg)	
				F2	OUTER THIGH (no 1)	
				F2	LYING QUADS (I each side)	
				F2	LYING HAMSTRINGS	
					(I each side)	
WEDNESDAY						
THURSDAY		S1	UPPER BACK	F2	ABDOMINALS (1)	10 MINS
		S1	CHEST	F1	ABDOMINALS (3)	
		S1	BICEPS	F1	BACK	
		S2	PULL DOWN (I on each side)	F2	INNER THIGH (I each leg)	
		S2	TRICEPS (I on each side)	F2	OUTER THIGH (no 2)	
FRIDAY	20 MINS					20 MINS
SATURDAY						
SUNDAY	20 MINS	S1	UPPER BACK	F2	ABDOMINALS (1)	30 MINS
		S1	CHEST	F2	ABDOMINALS (2)	
		S1	BICEPS	F1	BACK	
		S2	PULL DOWN (I each side)	F2	INNER THIGH (I each leg)	
		S2	TRICEPS (I each side)	F2	OUTER THIGH (I each leg)	

DON'T FORGET TO STRETCH !

WEEK NO:2 **YOUR BODY PLAN**

C = CHAIR   F = FLOOR   S = STANDING

DAY	WALKING	SETS	UPPER BODY	SETS	LOWER BODY	TOTAL TIME
MONDAY						
TUESDAY						
WEDNESDAY						
THURSDAY						
FRIDAY						
SATURDAY						
SUNDAY						

DON'T FORGET TO STRETCH !

WEEK NO:3 **SUGGESTED BODY PLAN**

C = CHAIR   F = FLOOR   S = STANDING

DAY	WALKING	SETS	UPPER BODY	SETS	LOWER BODY	TOTAL TIME
MONDAY						
TUESDAY	20 MINS	S1	UPPER BACK	F2	ABDOMINALS (1)	30 MINS
		S1	CHEST	F2	ABDOMINALS (2)	
		S2	PULL DOWN (1 each side)	F1	ABDOMINALS (3)	
				F2	BACK	
				F2	INNER THIGH (each leg)	
				F2	OUTER THIGH (each leg)	
WEDNESDAY	20 MINS					20 MINS
THURSDAY		S1	UPPER BACK	F2	ABDOMINALS (1)	10 MINS
		S1	CHEST	F2	ABDOMINALS (2)	
		S2	PULL DOWN (1 each side)	F1	ABDOMINALS (3)	
				F2	BACK	
				F4	INNER THIGH (2 each leg)	
				F4	OUTER THIGH (2 each leg)	
FRIDAY						
SATURDAY	20 MINS	S2	BICEPS + lower body movement	F2	ABDOMINALS (1)	30 MINS
		S1	UPPER BACK + lower body movt	F2	ABDOMINALS (2)	
		S1	CHEST + lower body movement	F2	ABDOMINALS (3)	
				F2	BACK	
				S2	2 IN 1 BUMS/TRICEPS	
				F2	LYING QUADS (1 each side)	
				F2	LYING HAMSTRINGS (1 each side)	
SUNDAY						

DON'T FORGET TO STRETCH !

WEEK NO:3 **YOUR BODY PLAN**

C = CHAIR   F = FLOOR   S = STANDING

DAY	WALKING	SETS	UPPER BODY	SETS	LOWER BODY	TOTAL TIME
MONDAY						
TUESDAY						
WEDNESDAY						
THURSDAY						
FRIDAY						
SATURDAY						
SUNDAY						

DON'T FORGET TO STRETCH !

WEEK NO:4 **SUGGESTED BODY PLAN**

C = CHAIR F = FLOOR S = STANDING

DAY	WALKING	SETS	UPPER BODY	SETS	LOWER BODY	TOTAL TIME
MONDAY	20 MINS	S2	UPPER BACK + lower body movt	F2	ABDOMINALS (1)	30 MINS
		S2	CHEST + lower body movt	F2	ABDOMINALS (2)	
				F4	ABDOMINALS (3)	
				F2	BACK	
TUESDAY						
WEDNESDAY		S2	PULL DOWN + lower body movt	F4	ABDOMINALS (1)	10 MINS
		S2	BICEPS + lower body movt	F4	ABDOMINALS (2)	
				F2	ABDOMINALS (3)	
				F4	BACK	
				F2	2 IN 1 BUMS/TRICEPS	
THURSDAY	20 MINS					20 MINS
FRIDAY						
SATURDAY	20 MINS			F4	ABDOMINALS (1)	30 MINS
				F4	ABDOMINALS (2)	
				F4	ABDOMINALS (3)	
				F4	BACK	
				F2	BELOW THE BELT KILLER	
					COMBO (1 on each leg)	
				F2	LYING QUADS (1 on each leg)	
SUNDAY						

DON'T FORGET TO STRETCH !

WEEK NO:4 **YOUR BODY PLAN**

C = CHAIR   F = FLOOR   S = STANDING

DAY	WALKING	SETS	UPPER BODY	SETS	LOWER BODY	TOTAL TIME
MONDAY						
TUESDAY						
WEDNESDAY						
THURSDAY						
FRIDAY						
SATURDAY						
SUNDAY						

DON'T FORGET TO STRETCH !

WEEK NO:5 **SUGGESTED BODY PLAN**

C = CHAIR   F = FLOOR   S = STANDING

DAY	WALKING	SETS	UPPER BODY	SETS	LOWER BODY	TOTAL TIME
MONDAY	20 MINS	S1	UPPER BACK + lower body movt	S2	2 IN 1 BUMS/TRICEPS	30 MINS
		S1	CHEST + lower body movt	F4	ABDOMINALS (1)	
				F4	ABDOMINALS (3)	
				F2	BACK	
				F2	OUTER THIGH (3)	
				F2	INNER THIGH	
TUESDAY						
WEDNESDAY	20 MINS			F4	ABDOMINALS (1)	30 MINS
				F4	ABDOMINALS (2)	
				F4	ABDOMINALS (3)	
				F4	BACK	
				F2	OUTER THIGH (3)	
				S2	INNER THIGH	
THURSDAY						
FRIDAY	20 MINS					20 MINS
SATURDAY						
SUNDAY		S1	UPPER BACK + lower body movt	F4	LYING QUADS (2 on each side)	10 MINS
		S1	CHEST + lower body movt	F2	KILLER COMBOS	
		S2	BICEPS + lower body movt	F2	ABDOMINALS (1)	
		S2	PULL DOWNS + lower body movt	F2	ABDOMINALS (2)	
				F2	ABDOMINALS (3)	
				F2	BACK	

DON'T FORGET TO STRETCH !

WEEK NO:5 **YOUR BODY PLAN**

C = CHAIR   F = FLOOR   S = STANDING

DAY	WALKING	SETS	UPPER BODY	SETS	LOWER BODY	TOTAL TIME
MONDAY						
TUESDAY						
WEDNESDAY						
THURSDAY						
FRIDAY						
SATURDAY						
SUNDAY						

DON'T FORGET TO STRETCH !

WEEK NO:6 **SUGGESTED BODY PLAN**

C = CHAIR   F = FLOOR   S = STANDING

DAY	WALKING	SETS	UPPER BODY	SETS	LOWER BODY	TOTAL TIME
MONDAY						
TUESDAY	20 MINS			S2	2 IN 1 BUMS/HAMS	30 MINS
				F4	LYING QUADS (I on each side)	
				F4	ABDOMINALS (1)	
				F4	ABDOMINALS (2)	
				F4	ABDOMINALS (3)	
				F4	BACK	
				F4	OUTER THIGH (3)	
				S4	INNER THIGH	
WEDNESDAY						
THURSDAY	20 MINS	S2	UPPER BACK + lower body movt	S2	2 IN 1 BUMS/HAMS	30 MINS
		S2	CHEST + lower body movt	F2	LYING QUADS	
		S4	PULL DOWNS + lower body movt	F4	ABDOMINALS (1)	
				F4	ABDOMINALS (2)	
				F4	ABDOMINALS (3)	
				F4	BACK	
FRIDAY						
SATURDAY	20 MINS			F4	KILLER COMBOS	30 MINS
				F2	LYING QUADS (I on each side)	
				F4	ABDOMINALS (1)	
				F4	ABDOMINALS (2)	
				F4	ABDOMINALS (3)	
				F4	BACK	
				S4	INNER THIGH	
				F2	OUTER THIGH (3)	
				F2	OUTER THIGH (2)	
SUNDAY						

DON'T FORGET TO STRETCH !

WEEK NO:6 **YOUR BODY PLAN**

C = CHAIR   F = FLOOR   S = STANDING

DAY	WALKING	SETS	UPPER BODY	SETS	LOWER BODY	TOTAL TIME
MONDAY						
TUESDAY						
WEDNESDAY						
THURSDAY						
FRIDAY						
SATURDAY						
SUNDAY						

DON'T FORGET TO STRETCH !

THE WALKING PROGRAMME

10 GOOD REASONS TO WALK

To help burn off stored energy (body fat) you need aerobic exercise. Walking is the perfect answer.

You should aim to walk briskly (as in really 'MOVE IT') for twenty minutes three times a week.

YES! YOU DO HAVE TIME

- It's cheap.
- It's easy.
- You know how to do it.
- It helps reduce stress.
- It's good for your heart and lungs.
- It helps improve bone density.
- It helps inch loss.
- No age barriers.
- Low risk of injury.
- You can go when and where you want – have legs, will travel.

- Walk to work.
- Walk to the shops.
- Walk the dog.
- Walk the kids.
- Walk for fun.

HOW DO I KNOW IF I'M WORKING HARD ENOUGH?

The simplest way of calculating how hard you are working is something called the 'rate of perceived exertion', or RPE for short. This is a useful option when 'on the go' as it does not require stop watches, heart rate charts or any specialized equipment. Quite simply, it is how you feel when exercising.

Rate of perceived exertion	
HOW HARD?	RATING
Very, very light	6, 7, 8
Very light	9, 10
Fairly light	11, 12
Fairly hard	13, 14
Hard	15, 16
Very hard	17, 18
Extremely hard	19

Another way to check your work level while walking is the Talk Test. If you can carry on a slightly breathless conversation while walking, then you are probably exercising at the right pace!

Progressing

After a week or so you should aim to:

**Increase your pace OR
Try walking up hills or slopes OR
Change what you walk on (no, I
don't mean your hands!), e.g.
sand, grass, gravel, etc.**

FACT 1

If the weather is very hot or
humid or windy it will increase
the demands on your body =
harder work due to external
factors

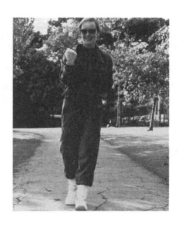

Progression chart

WEEK	HOW MANY TIMES PER WEEK	HOW LONG EACH TIME	RPE
1	x3	20 minutes	11–12
2	x2	20 minutes	11–12
	x1	20 minutes	13–14
3	x1	20 minutes	13–14
	x2	20 minutes	15–16
4	x2	20 minutes	13–14
	x1	20 minutes	15–16
5	x2	20 minutes	15–16
	x1	20 minutes	17–18
6	x2	20 minutes	17–18
	x1	20 minutes	19

This chart is a suggestion only, and shows a gentle, steady increase in
how hard you are working over the six-week programme.

Don't make the mistake of trying to progress too quickly. You will get no benefit and may very well injure yourself. Increase the level of difficulty by changing only one component at a time. For instance, increase your speed OR walk uphill today, but not both.

Your body will tell you if you are pushing it too hard. If it tells you any of the following, slow down; stop and check with your doctor immediately:

- pain or tightness in your chest
- sickness or nausea
- racing pulse
- dizziness
- exhaustion
- gasping for breath.

Listen to what your body says!

THE IMPORTANCE OF WATER

Carry a water bottle with you when you are exercising and make sure that you drink at regular intervals – little sips, often, are best.

You will be surprised at how much you will sweat when walking (provided you are working at the correct RPE), and dehydration will not allow you to exercise efficiently. If you prolong dehydration, it can lead to a variety of unwanted health symptoms so KEEP SLURPING!

WHAT TO WEAR?

- Good supportive flat walking boots or shoes, with cotton or wool socks for absorbency.
- Layers of clothing are best so that in cold weather you ADD layers, and in warm weather you SUBTRACT layers.
- If the weather is very cold a hat is a good idea. In wet weather a 'breathable' waterproof is a good investment.
- If you are walking in areas with a lot of pollution, a mask is a must.

SAFETY CHECKLIST

1 Walk in a group, or with a friend if you can.

2 Try to walk in daylight.

3 Carry a personal alarm.

4 If you are going to walk alone, tell someone where you are going and how long you will be.

5 Don't get lost!

6 Don't carry valuables, or wear jewellery.

7 Never walk wearing a personal stereo – you can't hear cars, would-be attackers or the dinner gong.

8 Walk tall in a confident manner.

9 Do not walk too closely to buildings, alley ways, or stationary vehicles.

10 Vary your route.

Did you know?
It has been estimated that even with no changes in your diet, if you walk for 45 minutes 4 times per week, you can lose 1½ pounds of body fat per month

WARMING UP
FOR WALKING

Use the first few minutes of your walk to 'warm up'. This means setting a gentle pace to ease your body into the exercise. Walk until you feel warm. Follow this 'warm up' with this series of stretches. It is important to do these stretches after your initial warm-up walk to avoid injury and get the maximum benefit. (Don't be embarrassed about doing these stretches outside!)

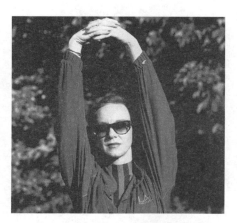

Overhead stretch

▶ Clasp hands, keeping elbows slightly bent

▶ Raise arms above your head, and push arms gently back

▶ HOLD for 8–16 counts

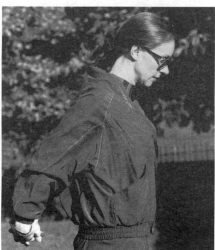

Shoulder stretch

▶ Clasp hands behind your back

▶ Keep elbows bent

▶ Slowly push hands upwards

▶ HOLD for 8–16 counts

Hamstring and calf stretch

▶ Bend one knee and place both hands on it

▶ Extend the other leg and push tailbone backwards, keeping your foot flat to the ground, and your knee 'soft'

▶ HOLD for 8–16 counts (each side)

▶ Now stretch your calf muscles by raising your toes (see photo)

▶ HOLD for 8–16 counts (each side)

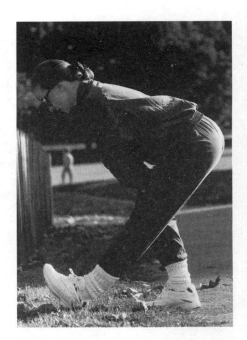

Shin stretch

▶ Hold on to a fence or wall

▶ Take toe behind and gently press down, taking care to keep your body weight over the supporting leg

▶ HOLD for 8–16 counts (each side)

▶ Repeat other side

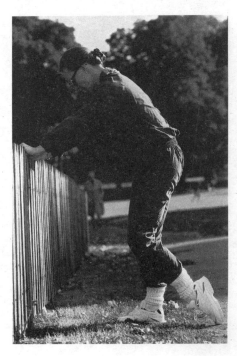

Quad stretch

▶ Hold on to a fence or wall

▶ Bend supporting leg slightly

▶ Bend the other leg and hold foot on top of shoe laces

▶ HOLD for 8–16 counts (each side)

Hip flexor stretch

▶ Hold on to a fence or wall

▶ Place one foot forward

▶ Place the other back, keeping your body weight over the ball of your back foot

▶ Slowly tilt pelvis forwards

▶ HOLD for 8–16 counts (each side)

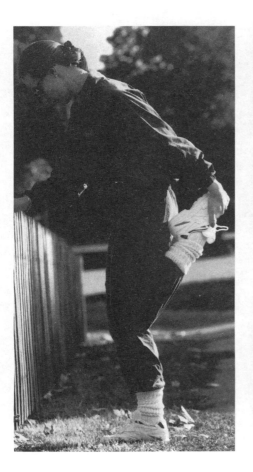

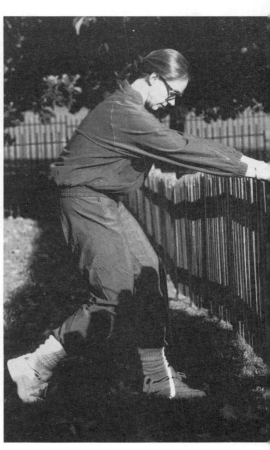

WALKING TECHNIQUE

Foot roll

Take care to place your feet correctly while walking. Take long strides, swinging from your hips and make sure that you work through the whole foot with each stride, so that the initial impact of each foot landing is taken on the heel, and you 'push off' from the ball of the foot.

Arm swing

To gain the maximum benefit from your walk, you must make sure that your arms swing freely from the shoulders. Really 'pump' your arms, driving the elbows back.

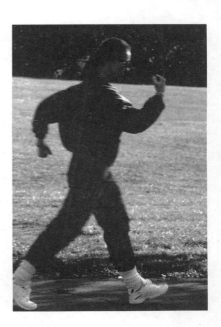

COOLING DOWN AFTER WALKING

When you finish your walk, if you are not going to follow it immediately with a band workout, you need to repeat all of the stretches shown on pages 37–39 for the warm-up. If you intend to go straight into a band workout you need only do a shin stretch (see page 38) and the following calf stretch. These calf and shin stretches are important as they are not included in the cool-down programme after the toning exercises using the Flex-a-Band.

Calf stretch

▶ Find a step or kerb

▶ Place the ball of one foot on the edge of the step

▶ Keeping the weight well forwards, over the supporting leg, slowly lower the heel an inch or so

▶ HOLD for 8–16 counts (each side)

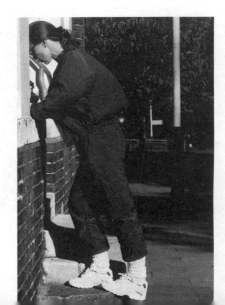

USING THE FLEX-A-BAND

THE HISTORY OF THE FLEX-A-BAND

Until recently the magical effects of latex rubber resistive training strips (commonly known as Flex-a-Band) have been confined to the medical profession (where they are called Cliniband), where spectacular results have been achieved in rehabilitation and physiotherapy departments.

Obviously, safety in these circumstances is of prime importance and here again, with correct use, the band comes out tops.

I have been using Flex-a-Bands since 1989 in normal fitness classes and also for personal training and remedial exercise classes for the elderly. The bands come in four different strengths, which are colour coded:

▶ FUSCHIA – light resistance

▶ JADE – medium resistance

▶ VIOLET – heavy resistance

▶ GOLD – extra heavy resistance.

For the majority of classes I use jade bands, as you can always increase resistance by tightening the band a little should you want to work harder. The only exception is when I work with pregnant or elderly clients when I use a lighter band; normally a jade band will be fine for most people. You will find one included with this book.

TAKING CARE OF YOUR FLEX-A-BAND

With normal use and correct care your Flex-a-Band should last for many months.

To make sure of this, do keep your band away from direct sunlight and heat, avoid contact with hand creams and rubs and take care not to pierce the band with sharp fingernails or jewellery – it's a good idea to take your rings off before you start using the band. Store the Flex-a-Band untied and sprinkled with a little talcum powder.

Beware if your training shoes have a heavily serrated sole as this can tear the band when you are performing an exercise with the band underneath one foot.

HOW TO HOLD THE BAND

▶ You can either wrap the band around your hands

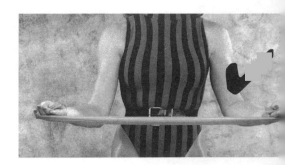

▶ OR simply hold it a few inches from each end

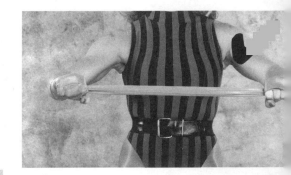

REMEMBER
The closer together your hands are, the greater the resistance will be

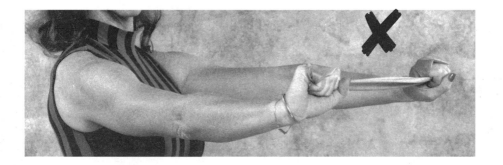

Do not allow your hands to 'turn back'.

Keep your wrist in line with the forearm.

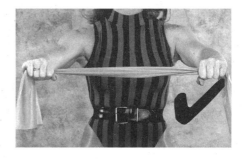

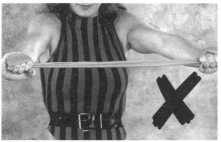

Watch out that you do not 'hunch' your shoulders when working the upper body.

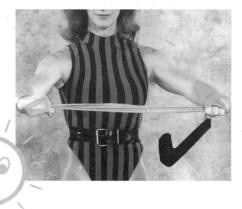

HOW TO TIE THE BAND

Always tie the band in a half loop or bow during exercise, as this will stop it pulling into a knot you cannot undo.

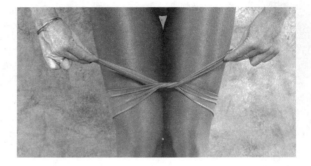

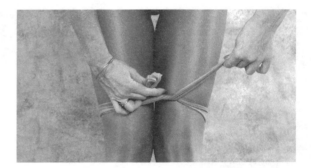

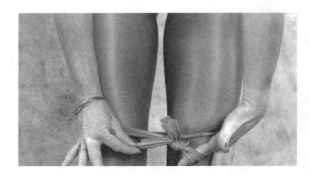

To untie, simply pull one end.

SAFETY AND TECHNIQUE

For your safety there are a few points to remember:

- Always check the band against the light for nicks or tears, as these can cause the band to snap while in use
- When working the upper body, keep your shoulders relaxed and down
- Always be aware of 'the line of pull'
- Relax the trapezius[1] muscles in between repetitions when working the upper body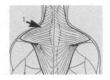
- Keep your wrist in line with the forearm when working the upper body
- Work your muscles through their fullest range
- Try to keep the band at its normal width when you are using it, as this will prevent it digging into your body or riding up
- Watch out if you have hairy legs – the band will provide instant depilation! Wear tights or tracksuit bottoms
- Don't over extend or 'lock' your joints
- Remember, do not try and rush this programme in a 'get fit quick' mad dash, e.g. on Tuesday morning trying to cram everything into the next few days because you have a hot date or special occasion on Friday night
- Always control the outward and inward movement of the band (i.e. don't pull out and then let it 'twang' back.

WHEN TO AVOID EXERCISING WITH THE BAND (OR CONTRA-INDICATIONS)

- If you have high blood pressure
- If you are pregnant
- If you suffer from RSI (Repetitive Strain Injury)
- If you have varicose veins
- If you have a history of shoulder injury or dislocation
- If you have had recent surgery
- If you are taking antibiotics.

If you have a history of knee problems always work with the band tied above the knees, taking care that the band does not rest on the kneecap.

REMEMBER

Rome wasn't built in a day, and if it had it would probably have fallen down the next!

WARMING UP FOR TONING

If you have not walked for twenty minutes before you do your body toning, you need to warm up your muscles ready for action. Do this for about five minutes; you should feel 'warm' at the end.

1

Start off by marching on the spot

2

Add shoulder shrugs while marching

3

Turn the shoulder shrugs into arm swings

4

Continue doing the same thing, but lift your knees up so that your thighs are parallel to the ground as you march

5

Keep at it, but instead of swinging your arms, make 'chest presses' as you march – bringing your arms together across your chest so that the elbows touch (take a look at the arm position in the exercise on page 79 too)

6

Return the arms to swinging position, and instead of bringing your knees high, walk so that you bring your heels up to your bum (hamstring curls)

7

Add upper back squeezes to this – moving your shoulders back as you walk

8

Cool down by walking on the spot swinging your arms, slowly gradually to a stop.

Always warm up either by using the walking programme, or the above warm-up before doing either the chair or toning exercises. After warming up, gently stretch the muscles you have just been using by following the exercises starting on page 83.

FIRM 'N' FIT WHILE YOU SIT

This chapter gives step-by-step instructions of exercises for the abdominal (stomach region), leg and upper body muscles. As they are all chair-based exercises, they are a great starting point, especially if you are unused to exercise. You can even do them in front of the TV! Try them for a few days at the start of your programme. After no more than two weeks you should find you are able to progress on to the Terrific Toning exercises.

Before starting these exercises, make sure you have:

● read the chapter on Using the Flex-a-Band

● warmed up, either by walking for twenty minutes and stretched your muscles (see pages 37– 39)

● or by marching on the spot, as described on page 46, and stretched your muscles (see pages 83 on).

You will need a straight-backed chair with a firm, flat seat (a dining room chair should be okay), and take care to sit up very straight on your 'bum bones'.

Watch out for the Body Check boxes to help you with the correct alignment. Look at the photographs carefully – they show the correct positions and also common errors.

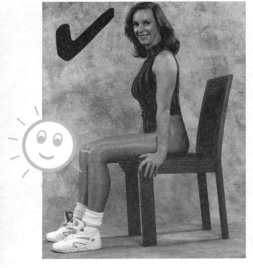

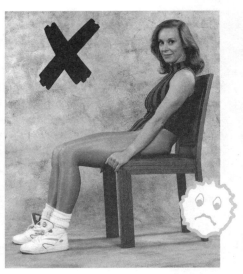

For inner thighs and abdominal work, a firm, solid foam-filled cushion is helpful. Even better is a child's sponge football; in fact, the resistance of the foam rubber football will produce the best results.

Each exercise includes a box which tells you:

● which movement to do on each count

● how many repetitions of each movement you should do to perform the exercise

● how many sets of the complete exercise you should try to do – start at the lower number and build up gradually.

Don't forget to keep a record of the exercises you do each day on the Body Plan chart on pages 22 – 23, and to measure your progress on the Figure Fact chart on page 21.

At the end of this chapter is a section on stretching your muscles after they have been worked. It is important to cool down in this way after every exercise session. These same stretching exercises will be used after the Terrific Toning exercises detailed in the next chapter.

While you are working through this programme, you may want to pay more attention to what you eat. Turn to the Food File on pages 89– 93 for some tips and guidelines on healthier eating.

ABDOMINALS

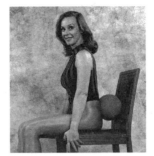

▶ Sit well forward and place the cushion or football between the base of your spine and the back of the chair

▶ Slowly push the base of your spine towards the back of the chair so that you squash the cushion or ball; exhale slowly

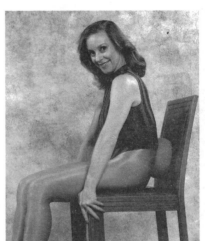

▶ Imagine that someone has punched you in the stomach – a bit drastic, but the body alignment should be easy to achieve)

▶ Release and inhale slowly as you straighten up

BODY CHECK

Take care not to lean back from the hips, or allow the shoulders to move back

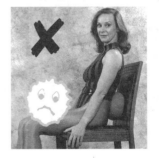

COUNTS	MOVE	REPETITIONS	SETS
1, 2, 3, 4	Squash ball/cushion	x8	2–4
5, 6, 7, 8	Release		

LEGS

Inner thigh

▶ Keeping feet flat on the floor, place the cushion or football between your knees

▶ Keeping your body slightly forwards, squeeze your knees together and squash the ball or cushion

▶ Release

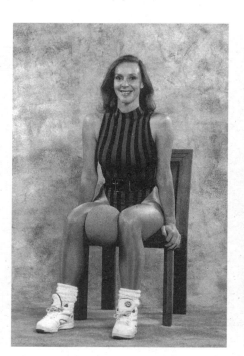

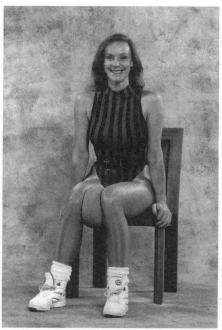

COUNTS	MOVE	REPETITIONS	SETS
1, 2, 3, 4	Squash ball/cushion	x8	2–4
5, 6, 7, 8	Release		

Outer thigh

▶ Tie the Flex-a-Band above your knees in a half bow

▶ Sitting forward on the chair, place your feet flat on the floor, a little wider than hip width apart; keep knees together

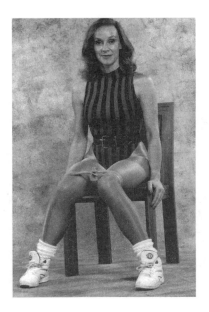

▶ Keeping back straight and stomach pulled in, push your knees as far apart as you can

▶ Release (don't allow your knees to 'ping' back – maintain the tension in the band on both inward and outward movements)

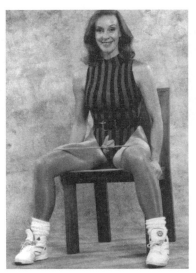

COUNTS	MOVE	REPETITIONS	SETS
1, 2, 3, 4	Push knees apart	x8	2–4
5, 6, 7, 8	Bring knees together		

Quadriceps (front of thigh)

▶ Place the band flat underneath the arch of your foot (make sure that you keep the foot flexed)

▶ Hold each end of the band tightly

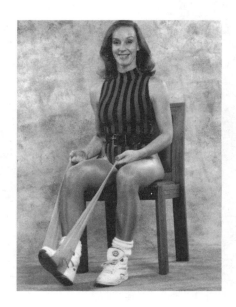

▶ Keeping your back straight, slowly extend your leg forward, leading with the heel

▶ Release

▶ Repeat with other leg

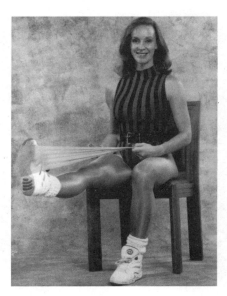

COUNTS	MOVE	REPETITIONS	SETS
1, 2, 3, 4	Extend leg	x8	1-2 on each leg
5, 6, 7, 8	Slowly lower leg		

Hamstrings (back of thigh)

▶ Keeping well forward on the chair (take care not to tip it over), tie the band around your ankles

▶ Keep your feet parallel and flat to the floor

▶ Slowly slide one foot back along the floor, feeling the back of the thigh contract (the foot should be underneath the chair as you finish sliding it backwards)

▶ Release by sliding the same foot forward again

▶ Repeat with other leg

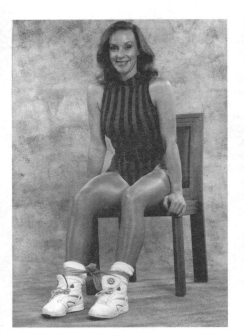
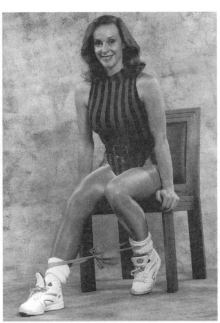

If you have knee problems try placing the sponge football in the crook of your knee and then drawing your foot back under the chair to squash the ball. Release and repeat.

COUNTS	MOVE	REPETITIONS	SETS
1, 2, 3, 4	Slide foot back	x8	1-2 on each leg
5, 6, 7, 8	Slide foot forward		

UPPER BODY

Nearly all of these upper body exercises shown can be done standing as well as using a chair as shown in the photographs. Choose whichever position you feel to be most comfortable.

Biceps

▶ Sitting straight with one foot slightly forward, place the band in the crook of the knee and hold both ends tightly

▶ Slowly pull your fists towards your shoulders

▶ Release

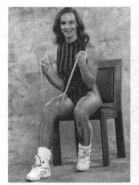
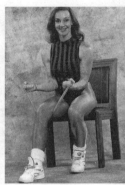

COUNTS	MOVE	REPETITIONS	SETS
1, 2, 3, 4	Pull fists towards shoulders	x8	1-2
5, 6, 7, 8	Maintaining tension, release		

Triceps

▶ Sit tall and wrap the band around your hands

▶ Take one hand to the opposite shoulder

▶ Keeping your shoulders down and relaxed, and your wrist in line with the forearm, slowly extend your arm to the side

▶ Repeat with the other arm

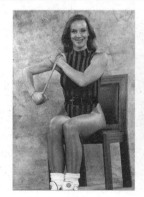
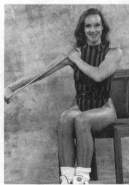

BODY CHECK

The upper arm should be lower than the shoulder when extended

COUNTS	MOVE	REPETITIONS	SETS
1, 2, 3, 4	Press fist away from body	x8	2-4 each side
5, 6, 7, 8	Release, maintaining tension		

Pull down

▶ Wrap the band around your hands

▶ Raise your arms above your head, keeping the band in your line of vision

▶ Keep the overhead arm absolutely steady

Take care not to allow your arms to go behind your head

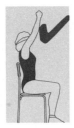 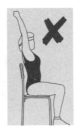

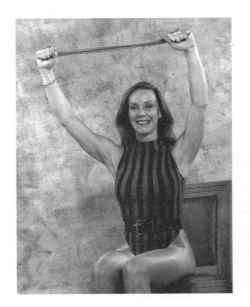

▶ Slowly pull down with your working arm aiming the elbow to the side of your waist

▶ Take care not to allow your body to drop to the side as you pull down

▶ Release

▶ Repeat on other side

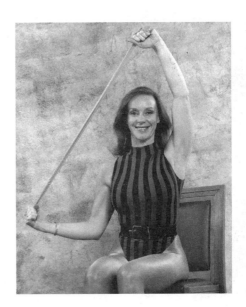

COUNTS	MOVE	REPETITIONS	SETS
1, 2, 3, 4	Pull elbow to waist	x8	2–4 each side
5, 6, 7, 8	Release		

Chest press

▶ Place the band flat across your
  shoulder blades and hold the ends
  tightly (the band should be taut)

▶ Push your arms forwards in a 'double
  punch' action – the arms should be at
  shoulder level

▶ Release

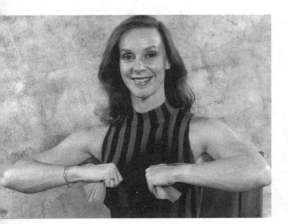
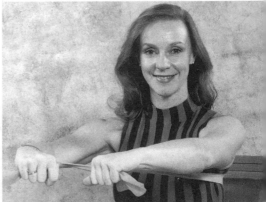

COUNTS	MOVE	REPETITIONS	SETS
1, 2, 3, 4	Push arms forward	x8	2–4
5, 6, 7, 8	Release		

TERRIFIC TONING

You should progress to this section after **no more than two weeks** on the Firm 'n' Fit While You Sit section – the quicker you build up your muscle strength, the quicker your body will start to show the results. Take a few moments to study the photographs and try out the exercises, to ensure you understand what you are meant to be doing.

I have given alternatives to the exercises so, for example, if you were not happy doing the lying side leg raises, you could do the outer thigh/hip exercise lying on your back.

As in the previous chapter, boxes are included after each exercise to prompt you:

● which movement to do on each count

● how many repetitions of each movement you should do to perform the exercise

● how many sets of the complete exercise you should try to do.

OUCH!

If your body says 'ouch!', don't continue. A warm, achy feeling is okay, but a sharp pain never is. Tune into your body, work hard and consistently but don't overdo it.

ABDOMINALS

These exercises require you to tie the Flex-a-Band above your knees. Before you tie the band above your knees, check that you are in the correct starting position.

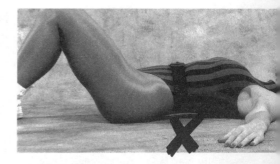

Do not allow your back to arch.

Contract your pelvic floor muscles. If you have difficulty finding the pelvic floor muscles (and they can be pretty elusive), practise by imagining trying to stop yourself in mid-flow while going to the loo!

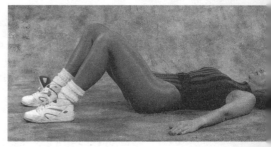

You do have to take care that your pelvic floor muscles stay taut. Pelvic floor muscles are notorious for 'taking a quick break' just as you get everything else right!

Turn to Using the Flex-a-Band (pages 41–45) to help you to tie the band correctly.

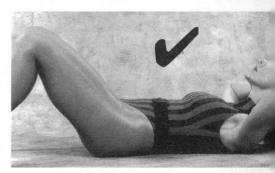

Clasp your hands at the base of your skull to support your head. This is the correct position for raising the upper body off the floor.

Take care not to allow your chin to drop into your chest. Imagine that you have a ball in between your chin and your collar bone.

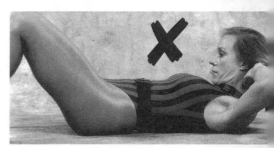

Do not move on until you are quite comfortable with this position

Abdominals 1 - Single crunch

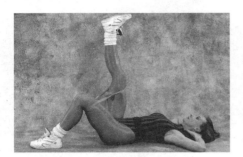
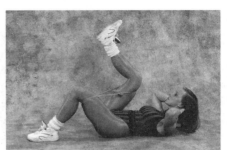

▶ Tie the band above your knees

▶ Lie flat on your back with one foot towards the ceiling keeping the knee slightly soft

▶ Bend the other leg, keeping the foot flat on the floor

▶ Maintaining good technique (pelvic floor taut and chin up), simultaneously raise the upper body off the floor while drawing the raised knee towards your shoulder

▶ Repeat with the other leg

COUNTS	MOVE	REPETITIONS	SETS
1, 2, 3, 4	Raise upper body and draw knee in (exhale)	x8–16 each leg	2–4
5, 6, 7, 8	Release (inhale)		

Abdominals 2 - Oblique crunch

▶ Lie flat on the floor

▶ Keeping the same elbow as working leg in contact with the floor, simultaneously take the opposite elbow towards the knee as you draw it in towards you

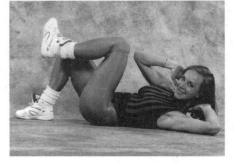

▶ Repeat with the other leg

COUNTS	MOVE	REPETITIONS	SETS
1, 2, 3, 4	Take opposite elbow to knee (exhale)	x8–16 each leg	2–4
5, 6, 7, 8	Release (inhale)		

Abdominals 3 – Reverse curl

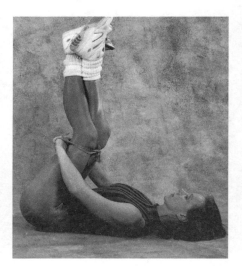

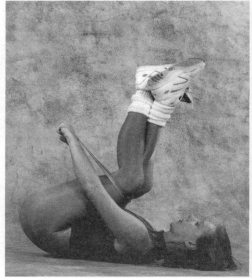

▶ Lie flat on the floor

▶ Raise both feet, with knees slightly bent, towards your shoulders (keep your tailbone on the floor and shoulders flat and relaxed)

▶ Place your hands through the band with the palms of your hands facing away from your body

▶ Push your hands away from your body as you draw your knees towards your shoulders (your tailbone should lift a few inches off the floor)

▶ This should be a controlled movement

You should try to do all the abdominal exercises one after another, e.g.:
1 set each side
single crunch – 2 x (sets of 8)
oblique crunch – 2 x (sets of 8)
reverse curl – 1x (set of 8)

Increase your repetitions and sets as you progress.
In between each set, pull your knees in towards your chest and relax for a count of 8.

COUNTS	MOVE	REPETITIONS	SETS
1, 2, 3, 4	Draw knees towards shoulders (exhale)	x8–16	1–2
5, 6, 7, 8	Release (inhale)		

Back strengthener (no band)

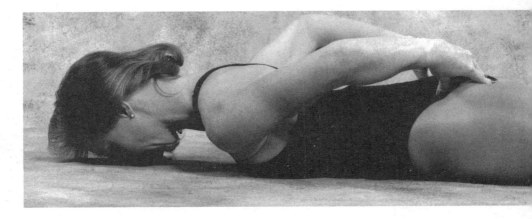

▶ Lie face down on the floor and place
  your fingertips just above your bum

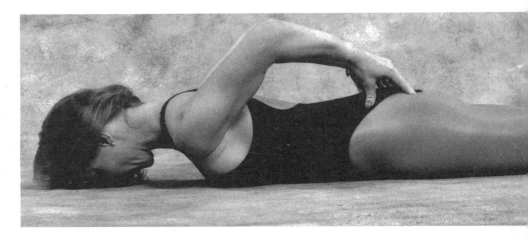

▶ Squeeze your elbows together

CONTINUED OVERLEAF...

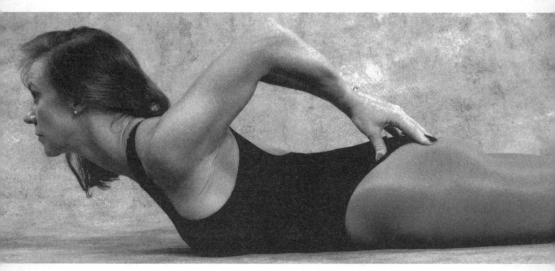

▶ Keeping your feet on the floor, raise
   your upper body

▶ Lower the upper body

▶ Release elbows

You will find that the lower back muscles
tire quite quickly. It is better to start with
only 1 set of 4 repetitions done well than
to try to start with 8 and do them badly.

COUNTS	MOVE	REPETITIONS	SETS
1	Squeeze elbows together	x4–8	1 –2
2	Raise upper body		
3	Lower upper body		
4	Release elbows and relax		

Inner thigh

Body check

This exercise is absolutely brilliant for targeting those 'squidgy' bits at the top of the inner thigh, but your starting body position is the key to making it work. Take a few moments to make sure that you are in the correct position.

Take care not to allow your hips to roll backwards. Keep your knees level and flex your feet. Don't bend your arm to place it under your head. Keep your arm extended along the floor and the other arm in front of your body for support. You should be able to see your toes as you look down your body.

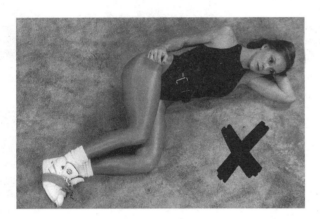

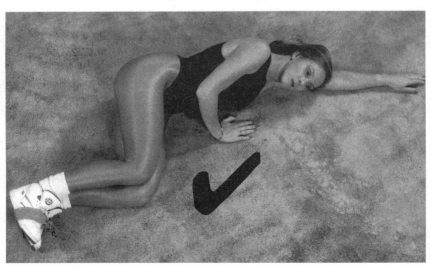

▶ Tie the band into approximately a 12"
  loop

▶ Place your feet into the band so that it is
  over the shoe laces of your top leg and
  under the arch of the foot of your bottom
  leg

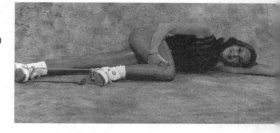

▶ Angle the bottom leg slightly forwards

▶ Draw the top leg towards your chest
  and hold under the knee

▶ Remember to keep your feet flexed
  otherwise the band will fly off!

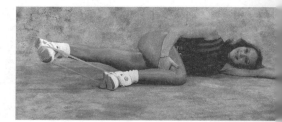

▶ Slowly raise the lower leg a few inches
  off the floor, with the inside of your heel
  towards the ceiling (if you lift the leg
  higher than a few inches you will lose
  your correct body placement)

▶ Take care not to twist, or 'sickle', your foot

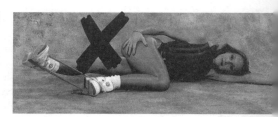

▶ Release – do not allow your leg to touch
  the floor between repetitions

▶ Repeat with other leg

As you become more proficient with this exercise try adding small 'pulsing' movements.
A 'pulse' movement is a small movement at the most difficult point of the exercise. In this
instance, the most difficult point is count 3, when the leg is raised at its highest point.

When you feel ready to add pulses, each time you reach this highest point, pulse the leg
4 times, then lower.

COUNTS	MOVE	REPETITIONS	SETS
1, 2, 3	Lift leg	x8 each leg	1–2
4	Lower (do not allow leg to rest on floor)		

Outer thigh/hips 1–on back

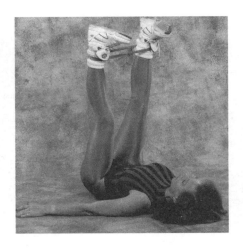

▶ With the band around your ankles, lie
flat on your back with the soles of your
feet towards the ceiling

▶ Your knees should be relaxed

▶ Keeping your toes turned in slightly,
pull your legs apart, hold and release

▶ Make sure you maintain the tension in
the band on both the outward and the
inward movements

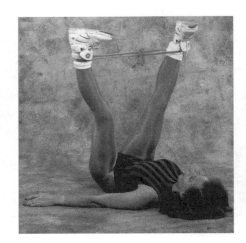

COUNTS	MOVE	REPETITIONS	SETS
1,	Pull legs apart	x8	2–4
2, 3	Hold		
4	Release		

Outer thigh/hips 2 – Prone

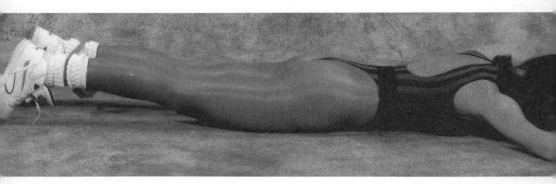

▶ Lie face down with the band tied
around your ankles and your forehead
resting on your hands

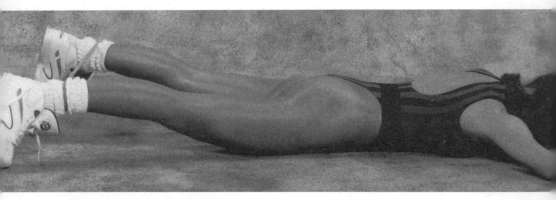

▶ Keeping your hips in contact with the
floor, slowly pull your legs apart and
release

COUNTS	MOVE	REPETITIONS	SETS
1	Pull legs apart	x8	2–4
2, 3	Hold		
4	Release		

Outer thigh/hips 3 - Seated

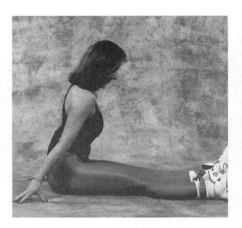

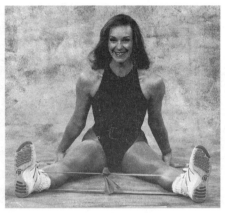

▶ Balancing on your 'bum bones', with the band tied around your ankles, sit very tall with your hands resting on the floor slightly behind you

▶ Keeping your back straight and shoulders slightly forwards, slowly pull your legs apart (keeping your knees flat)

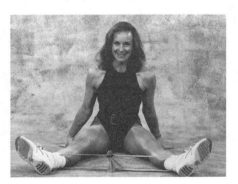

▶ Rotate both legs out from the hips – again, keeping your knees flat and your back straight

COUNTS	MOVE	REPETITIONS	SETS
1	Pull legs apart	x4–8	1–2
2	Rotate legs out		
3	Straighten legs		
4	Control move as you bring your legs together		

Lying quads

▶ Lean back on your elbows with the band underneath one foot

▶ Hold both ends tightly

▶ Keeping your ribcage lifted, slowly extend your working leg

▶ Release

▶ Repeat with other leg

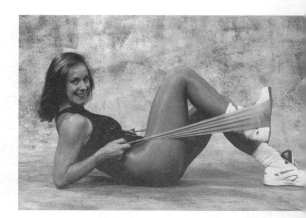

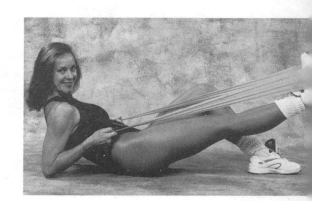

TIP

You may be more comfortable with a cushion or mat underneath your elbows

COUNTS	MOVE	REPETITIONS	SETS
1, 2	Extend leg	x8–16	2–4 each leg
3, 4	Release		

THE BELOW THE BELT KILLER COMBO

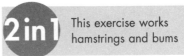

2 in 1 This exercise works hamstrings and bums

▶ Lie face down, with the band around one ankle and under the sole of the working foot

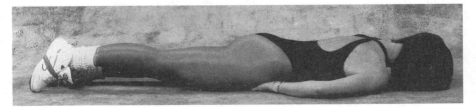

▶ Place your hands under your hip bones

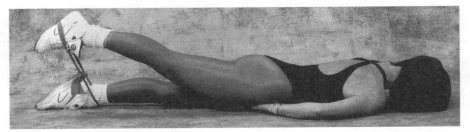

▶ Keeping your hip bones pressed into the palms of your hands, raise the working leg, keeping it straight

▶ Lower

Lying hamstrings

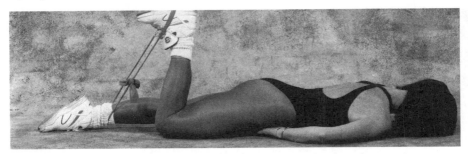

▶ In exactly the same starting position as before slowly squeeze the heel of the working leg as far as you can towards your bum

▶ Release

▶ Repeat these two exercises with the other leg, OR go on to the next exercise

Killer bum

This is a progression from the previous two exercises.

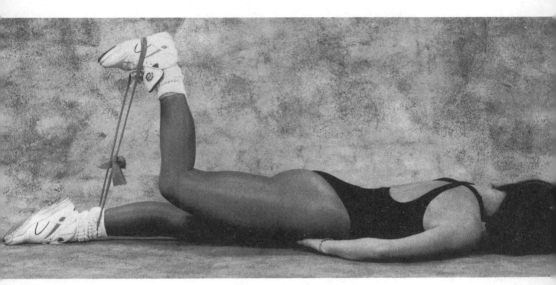

▶ Once you have squeezed your heel towards your bum,
  KEEPING BOTH HIP BONES TOUCHING YOUR HANDS
  press the heel of your working leg as far as you can
  towards the ceiling

▶ Release

▶ Repeat these three movements with the other leg

COUNTS	MOVE	REPETITIONS	SETS
1	Lift leg straight	x4–8	1 on each leg
2	Lower		
3	Squeeze heel to bum		
4	Press heel to ceiling		
5, 6	'Pulse'		
7	Straighten leg		
8	Lower		

**(if you manage to do more than one set on let me know and I'll give you
a medal – I can't!)**

Inner thigh (standing)

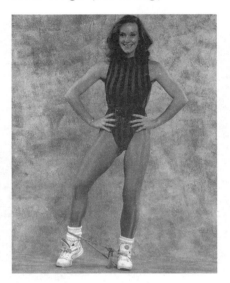

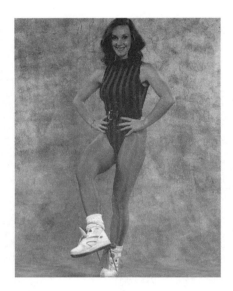

▶ Tie the band into approximately a 12"
loop

▶ Place the band underneath the
supporting foot and around the ankle of
the working leg

▶ Move the working leg across the
mid-line of your body

▶ Imagine that you are kicking a football
with the inside of your heel, but keep the
movement slow and
controlled, not jerky

▶ Release

▶ Repeat with the
other leg

▶ Do not allow your
working leg to twist

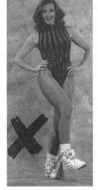

COUNTS	MOVE	REPETITIONS	SETS
1, 2	Push working leg across mid-line of body	x4–8 each leg	2–4
3, 4	Bring leg back and rest ball of foot on floor		

Outer thigh/hips (standing)

▶ Tie the band above your knees and transfer your body weight over the supporting leg

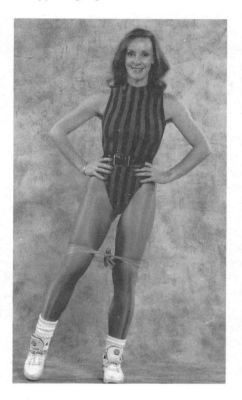 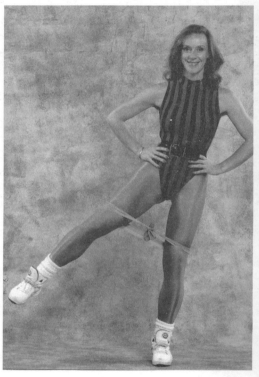

▶ Keeping your thighs parallel, lift your leg to the side taking care not to allow your body to lean

▶ Your foot should be slightly flexed

BODY CHECK
Keep abdominals tight, and knees slightly relaxed

▶ Watch out that you do not twist your body thereby allowing the supporting leg to 'roll' inwards and the working leg to rotate outwards (if you do this you will be working your quads and hip flexors instead of your outer thigh and hips, not to mention risking injury)

▶ Release

▶ Repeat with the other leg

A nice variation on this exercise is to add in 1 or 2 sets of 8 repetitions of alternate leg lifts.

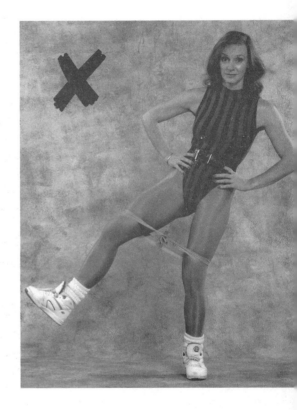

COUNTS	MOVE	REPETITIONS	SETS
1	Lift leg	x8	1–2 on each side
2	Lower leg		

Standing bums/hamstrings

▶ Place the band underneath the sole of the supporting foot, and around the ankle of your working leg

BODY CHECK
Keep your tummy tight and tailbone pulled down

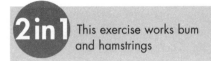

2 in 1 This exercise works bum and hamstrings

▶ Keeping your working leg straight, lift it a few inches off the floor

▶ Lower

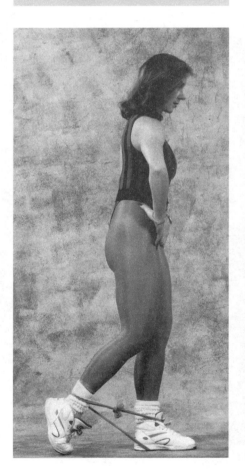

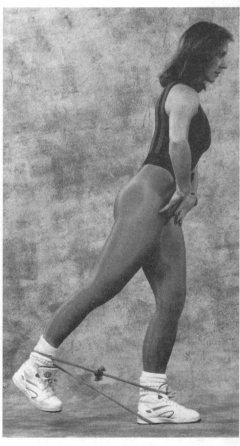

▶ Now squeeze the heel of your working leg towards your bum (it probably won't go far)

▶ Lower

▶ Repeat these two movements with the other leg

This exercise requires a lot of strength. If you haven't eaten your quota of spinach for the day à la Popeye, or you just can't do it, opt for a floor version or even a chair!

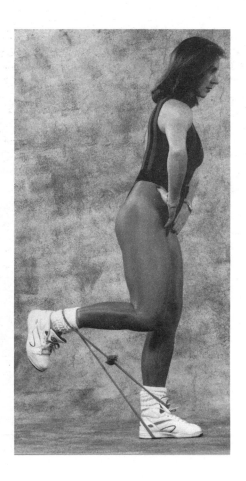

COUNTS	MOVE	REPETITIONS	SETS
1	Lift leg (straight)	x4–8	1 each leg
2	Lower		
3	Squeeze heel to bum		
4	Lower		

Bums (standing)

▶ Place your heel firmly on one end of the band and hold the other

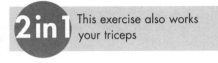

2 in 1 This exercise also works your triceps

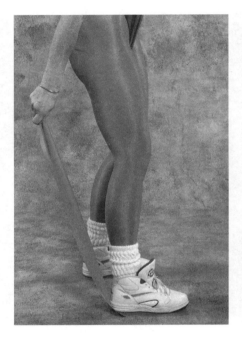

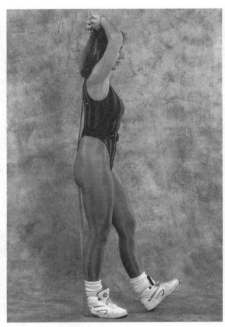

▶ Raise your front toes of your other foot to make sure that your weight stays over the other end of the band

▶ Take the band in both hands and hold it at the crown of your head

▶ Keeping your abdominals tight and pulled in, slowly bend your knees and push both hands towards the ceiling

BODY CHECK
Take care not to arch your back

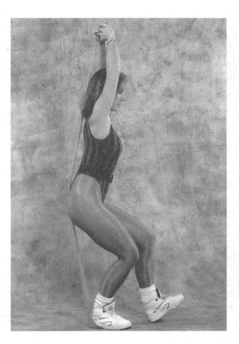

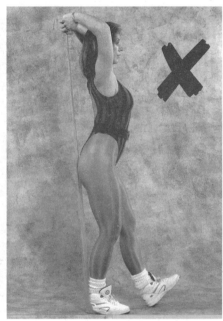

BODY CHECK
Keep your upper arms in line with your ears

▶ Release your arms and straighten your legs, squeezing hard into the bum muscles of your weight-bearing leg as you straighten

▶ Repeat with the other leg

COUNTS	MOVE	REPETITIONS	SETS
1, 2, 3, 4	Bend knees and push up arms	x8	2–4
5, 6, 7, 8	Release and straighten		

UPPER BODY

Upper back

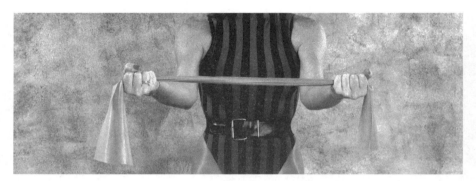

▶ Place the band flat across the palms of your hands

▶ Grip tightly

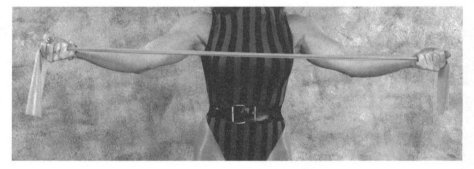

▶ Slowly pull your hands apart feeling your shoulder blades squeeze together

▶ Release (maintaining the tension in the band)

> **BODY CHECK**
> Keep your shoulders down and relaxed throughout this exercise

COUNTS	MOVE	REPETITIONS	SETS
1, 2	Pull hands apart	x4–8	1–2
3, 4	Release		
1	Pull hands apart		
2, 3, 4, 5, 6, 7	'Pulse'		
8	Release		

Chest

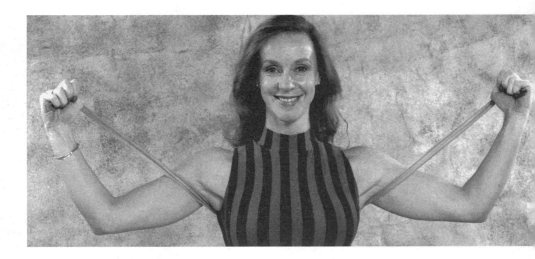

▶ Place the band flat across your shoulder blades; and bring it under both your arms and grip both ends tightly

▶ Slowly squeeze your forearms together in front of your face

▶ Release

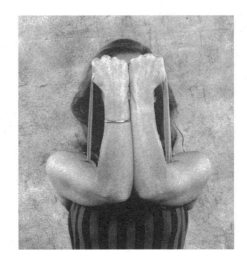

COUNTS	MOVE	REPETITIONS	SETS
1, 2	Squeeze arms together	x8	2–4
3. 4	Release		

Biceps

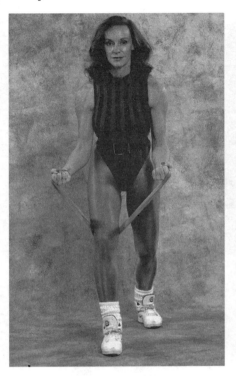

- Assume a split stance with one leg forwards and one back with your knees bent and your weight forwards over your front foot

- Place the band in the crook of the front knee (if the band does not feel secure, increase the degree of bend in the front leg)

- Hold both ends of the band firmly

- Squeeze both fists upwards towards your shoulders

BODY CHECK
Keep palms upwards

COUNTS	MOVE	REPETITIONS	SETS
1, 2, 3	Squeeze fists towards shoulders	x8	1-2
4	Release		
1	Squeeze fists towards shoulders		
2, 3, 4	Release		

Triceps

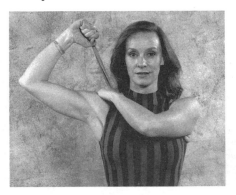

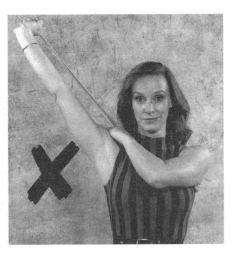

▶ Wrap the band around both hands

▶ Take one hand to the opposite
shoulder

▶ Press the hand of your working arm
upwards towards the ceiling

▶ Do not 'lock' the elbow joint, or allow
the hand to snap backwards

▶ Release

▶ Repeat with the other arm

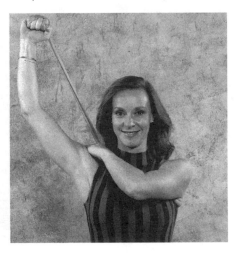

COUNTS	MOVE	REPETITIONS	SETS
1, 2, 3	Press hand upwards	x8	1–2
4	Release		
1	Press hand upwards		
2, 3, 4	Release		

TAKE IT TO THE MAX!?

To cram the most effort into the upper body work and get really fast overall results, keep the lower body moving while working the upper body; for instance, you could try marching on the spot while doing the upper back exercise, adding wide knee bends as you work your chest or adding split lunges to the biceps exercise.

COOLING DOWN

At the end of your band workout it is vital that you cool down by stretching the muscles you have been working. Work through the stretching exercises on pages 83–88.

STRETCHING

At the end of your band workout you must cool down by stretching the muscles that you have been working. Follow the instructions carefully and look at the photographs to check you are correctly aligned. Each stretch should be held for between eight and sixteen counts.

Hamstring stretch (level 1)

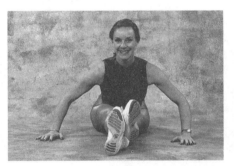

- Sit tall and cross your ankles, with your hands on the floor

- Keeping your ribcage lifted, slowly lean forwards, keeping your shoulders relaxed and down and your back flat.

Make sure you do both legs

- HOLD for 8–16 counts (each leg)

Hamstring stretch (level 2)

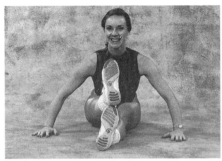

- As before, but place one heel on top of the toe underneath the foot, giving the hamstring a slightly stronger stretch

Outer thigh/hips

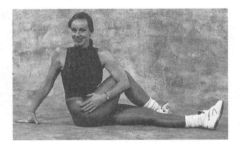

- Sit tall with legs outstretched in front of you

- Bend one leg over the other (the foot of the bent leg should be a little below the knee of the straight leg)

- Place the opposite arm along the outside of your thigh

- Place the other arm behind you for support

- Slowly and carefully rotate the upper body away from the bent foot

- HOLD for 8–16 counts (each side)

Inner thigh/groin

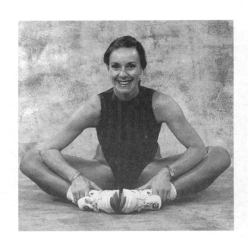

▶ Place the soles of your feet as close together as you can

▶ Hold your ankles, not your toes

▶ Press your elbows gently down on the inside of your knees as you lean forwards, keeping your back flat and your chin lifted

▶ HOLD for 8–16 counts

Waist

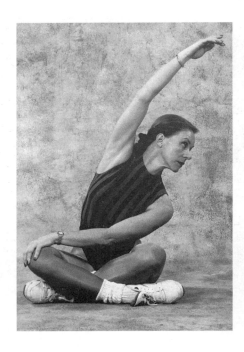

▶ Cross your legs (you should feel no discomfort in the knees or hips – if you do, move your feet forwards a little)

▶ Place one hand on the opposite knee

▶ Keeping both your bum bones on the floor, extend the other arm up and over, keeping the arm level with your ear

▶ HOLD for 8–16 counts (each side)

Hips

> **BODY CHECK**
> **Keep both bum bones on the floor**

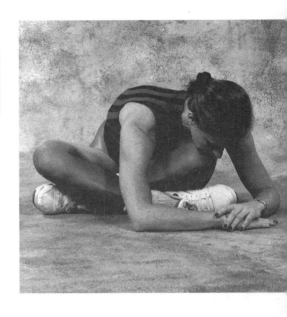

▶ Sit cross legged

▶ Lean forwards, aiming your chin to one knee

▶ Place your hands (or forearms, depending on your flexibility) on the floor either side of your knee

▶ HOLD for 8–16 counts (each side)

Upper back

▶ Give yourself a hug – you deserve it!

▶ HOLD for 8 –16 counts

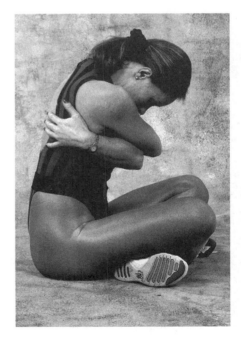

Chest

▶ Place your fingertips either side of the base of your spine

▶ Keep your shoulders down

▶ Squeeze your elbows together, feeling the stretch across your chest

▶ HOLD for 8–16 counts

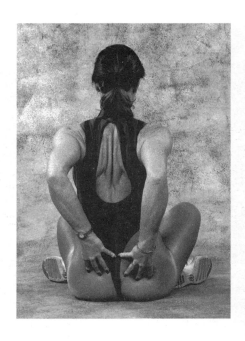

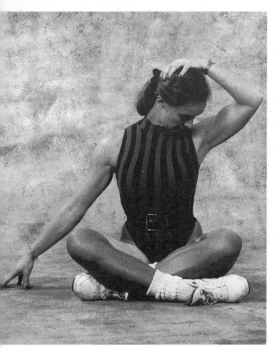

Neck and upper back

▶ Sit very tall on both bum bones

▶ Place the fingertips of one hand on the floor

▶ Place your other hand on the back of your head

▶ Turn your head towards your raised elbow and drop your chin, aiming your nose at your nipple

▶ HOLD for 8–16 counts (each side)

Triceps

▶ Try to touch the fingertips of both hands together behind your back

▶ Do not drop the upper body

▶ HOLD either position for 8–16 counts (each side)

If this is too much for you, gently stretch the triceps by taking your right hand to your right shoulder. Pressing your left hand to the triceps of your right arm try to aim your elbow towards the ceiling.

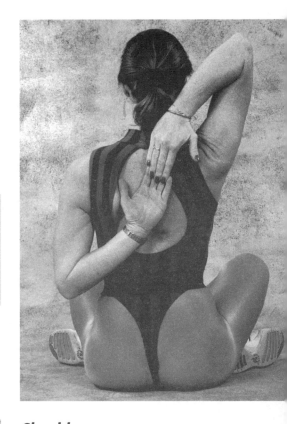

Shoulders

▶ Bring one arm across your body

▶ Keep both shoulders relaxed and down

▶ Place one hand just above your elbow

▶ HOLD for 8–16 counts (each side)

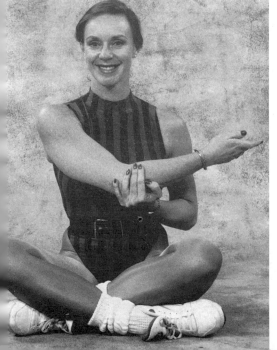

Quads

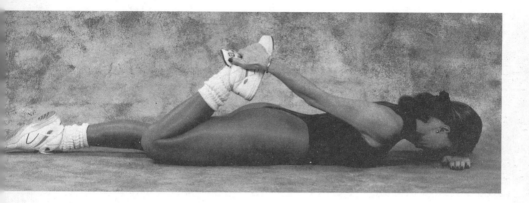

▶ Lie face down and rest your forehead
on one hand

▶ Bend the opposite leg

▶ With the other hand, hold on to the
top of your foot near your shoe laces

▶ HOLD for 8–16 counts each side

FOOD FILE

THE **7** NUTRIENTS ESSENTIAL FOR LIFE

▶ Carbohydrates – these give you the power to work your body, e.g. pasta, bread, rice, potatoes, bananas.

▶ Vitamins – these cannot be manufactured by the body, yet are required for growth, reproduction, repair and body maintenance.

▶ Fats – you need these to combine with other nutrients to form cell membranes, bile, vitamin D, blood lipids and steroids.

▶ Water – our most basic need.

▶ Fibre – this is not strictly a nutrient, but it is vital for better elimination and to decrease appetite.

▶ Minerals – essential factors in energy production, body building and maintenance.

▶ Proteins – the basic building blocks of the body's tissues.

Food for life checklist
If you are what you eat, and you eat too much saturated fat, guess what you'll be? Most saturated fat is found in animal products, i.e. dairy products and meat (see The Four Basic Food Groups on page 91. See the table or pages 92-93 for guidelines on how much fat typical foods contain). Some is found in certain vegetable oils, and in both hard and soft margarines.

✔ EAT LESS FAT

✔ TRY TO LIMIT YOUR SUGAR INTAKE
This means in cakes, biscuits and sweets, but also in drinks. Remember sugar contains calories and absolutely no nutrients.

✔ VARY YOUR FOOD TYPES
See The Four Basic Food Groups listed on page 91.

✔ WATCH OUT FOR 'THE DEMON DRINK'
Booze contains loads of calories, e.g. 275ml ($\frac{1}{2}$ pint) lager = 90 calories; 1 measure of any spirit = 50 calories (not including mixer); 140ml ($\frac{1}{4}$ pint) of wine = 90–140 calories, depending on whether it is dry white wine (= 90 calories), or sweet white wine (= 140 calories).
Women should try not to drink more than 14 units of alcohol per week (spread across the week).

1 UNIT OF ALCOHOL =

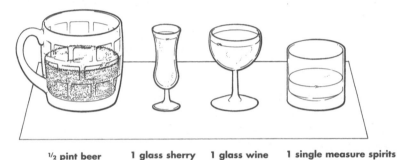

| $\frac{1}{2}$ pint beer | 1 glass sherry | 1 glass wine | 1 single measure spirits |

✔ TRY TO CUT BACK YOUR SALT INTAKE

✔ TRY TO EAT 2–5 PIECES OF FRESH FRUIT EACH DAY
It is best to eat fruit early in the day. If you eat fruit in the evening (especially fruits like apples and pears), they can have a tendency to 'ferment' in your stomach overnight, causing a nasty bloated feeling–YEUCH!

✔ EAT LOTS OF FIBRE-RICH AND STARCHY FOODS
Starchy foods (carbohydrates) tend to be filling without containing too many calories (take care not to add oily sauces or sugary toppings). Fibre is necessary for the reasons already stated.

✔ ENJOY YOUR FOOD

✔ DON'T OVER-COOK YOUR FOOD
This will destroy the vitamins and minerals it contains.

DID YOU KNOW?
Approximately 55–60 per cent of your daily calorie intake should be consumed as carbohydrate

✔ TRY TO INCLUDE ONE SMALL POT OF LIVE YOGHURT IN YOUR DAILY DIET
The ones that contain the live bifidus and acidophilus bacteria are best–sorry to get so technical; Loseley do good ones. The reason for this inclusion is that the live culture helps to maintain the balance of natural flora in the gut (I've probably just put you off it for life–sorry!).

✔ DRINK LOTS OF WATER
At least eight glasses per day.

THE **4** BASIC FOOD GROUPS

1 Milk/dairy products

2 Meat and other proteins

3 Fruits and vegetables

4 Grains/starchy foods.

Make sure your daily diet is a balance of these four.

HEALTHY EATING AND EASY WAYS TO REDUCE FAT

Simple changes in your eating habits to reduce your overall fat intake are very easy to make. You'll find that your own body fat will reduce without having to worry about special menus or weighing ingredients, which tend to be time-consuming, and frequently anti-social! Diets are temporary and the results tend to be temporary too. Have confidence in your own ability to make a difference to your own figure without being told exactly what to eat day by day. Think for yourself, and use the information in this book to help build yourself a beautiful body.

How much fat?

Below is a guide to how much fat some everyday foods contain. It is worth getting into the habit of checking food labels to see how much fat you are eating. As you can see from the table, some foods contain considerably more fat than others. For example, chicken with skin contains almost three times as much fat as chicken without skin. And just look at the difference between tuna in oil and tuna in brine!

FOOD	*Fat grams*
Dairy products	
MILK (1 pint)	
Gold Top	28.6 grams
Whole	22.0 grams
Semi-skimmed	9.0 grams
Skimmed	0.6 grams
CHEESE (per 60 grams)	
Cheddar	20.0 grams
Edam	14.0 grams
Low-fat Cheddar	8.0 grams
Very low-fat cottage cheese	0.2 grams
YOGHURT (per 100 grams)	
Low-fat plain	0.3 grams
Low-fat fromage frais	0.3 grams
'Live' low-fat (flavoured)	1.3 grams

FOOD	*Fat grams*
Poultry (per 100 grams)	
Roast duck (no skin)	9.7 grams
Roast chicken (no skin)	5.4 grams
Roast chicken (with skin)	14.0 grams
Roast turkey (no skin)	2.7 grams
Fats and oils (per 10 grams)	
Butter	8.0 grams
Margarine (all types)	8.0 grams
Low-fat spread	4.0 grams
Oil (all types)	10.0 grams
Meat (per 100 grams)	
Roast lamb	8.0 grams
Roast beef (lean)	9.0 grams
Roast pork (lean)	7.0 grams
1 large sausage	10.0 grams
Low-fat sausage	5.5 grams
Salami	45.2 grams
Pork pie	27.0 grams
Corned beef	12.1 grams
Liver sausage	26.9 grams
Fish (per 100 grams)	
Fried, battered cod	10.3 grams
Pilchards in tomato sauce	5.4 grams
Tuna (in oil)	22.0 grams
Tuna (in brine)	1.0 grams
Prawns	1.8 grams
Tinned salmon	8.2 grams
Smoked mackerel	15.5 grams
Steamed plaice	1.9 grams
Steamed trout	4.5 grams
Sweets and snacks	
Digestive biscuit	3.0 grams
Packet of crisps	9.0 grams
Packet of crisps (low fat)	7.0 gram
Small bag of peanuts	12.0 grams
Small chocolate bar	15.0 grams
Dairy ice cream (60g)	5.9 grams

ONE LAST WORD

You now have all the information that you need to succeed in achieving the Nine Hour New You.

If you miss a day or so of your workout plan, don't worry. Just pick up where you left off. At the end of the programme you'll still feel fitter, firmer – and above all confident about staying that way for ever. You'll never look back.

Remember the golden rules for achieving a healthy, shapely body:

- good nutrition
- exercise
- rest
- fresh air
- acceptance

Adopt a positive and peaceful approach to yourself, focus on what you know are your good points rather than what you might think are your worst, and be 'happy in your skin'. These are the ingredients for a new you – let me know how you get on!

Miranda Llewellyn
Body Magic
c/o Boxtree Limited
Broadwall House
21 Broadwall
London SE1 9PL

THE NINE HOUR NEW YOU
EXERCISES EASY REFERENCE

ARMS Chair/standing

Biceps	54/80
Triceps	54/81
2 in 1 Bums (standing) (with triceps)	76-77
Pull down	55

BACK Chair/standing

Upper back	78

Floor

Lower back (Back strengthener)	61-62

CHEST Chair/standing

Chest press	56
Chest	79

ABDOMINALS

Chair

Abdominals (chair)	49
Abdominals 1 (Single crunch)	59
Abdominals 2 (Oblique crunch)	59
Abdominals 3 (Reverse curl)	60

BUMS Floor

Below the Belt Killer Combo (Lying hamstrings & Killer bum)	
	69-70

Standing

2 in 1 Bums (standing) (with triceps)	76-77
2 in 1 Standing bums/hamstrings	74-75

LEGS

Inner thigh (sitting)	50
Inner thigh (lying)	63-64
Inner thigh (standing)	71
Outer thigh/hips (standing)	72-73

Chair

Outer thigh	51
Quadriceps (quads) (front of thigh)	52

Floor

Outer thigh/hips 1 - On back	65
Outer thigh/hips 2 - Prone	66
Outer thigh/hips 3 - Seated	67

Chair/floor

Lying quads	68

Chair

Hamstrings (back of thigh)	53

Floor

Below the Belt Killer Combo (Lying hamstrings & Killer bum)	
	69-70

Standing

2 in 1 Standing bums/hamstrings	74-75

FLEX·A·BAND is supplied by
Medisport International Ltd

The product is just one of a comprehensive
range of sports care products for the
prevention and treatment of sports injuries.
These products include everything from knee
and back supports to tennis elbow splints,
sportsbalm, ice packs, strapping tape and
blister patches. All are available through
Medisport Centres in high street pharmacies
and the major multiples. If you wish to
replace the Jade Flex-a-Band enclosed with
this book, ask your local pharmacy where
you see the sign, or telephone Medisport for
further information or details of your nearest
stockist.

Medisport International Ltd
Medisport House
Petersfield Business Park
Petersfield
Hampshire GU32 3QA
ENGLAND
Tel: 01730 231132
Fax: 01730 231777